D1650422

Simple Eye Diagnosis

HECTOR BRYSON CHAWLA
M.B. Ch.B. (St Andrews) F.R.C.S.E. D.O. (London)

Consultant Ophthalmic Surgeon, Royal Infirmary of Edinburgh, and former fellow in the Retina Service, Northwestern University, Chicago, U.S.A.

Second Edition

CHURCHILL LIVINGSTONE
EDINBURGH LONDON AND NEW YORK 1975

This book is dedicated to Dr J.F. Cullen, to whom I owe so much.

CHURCHILL LIVINGSTONE
Medical Division of Longman Group Limited

Distributed in the United States of America by Longman Inc., New York and by associated companies, branches and representatives throughout the world.

© Longman Group Limited 1973, 1975

First edition 1973
Second edition 1975

ISBN 0 443 01263 6

Library of Congress Catalog Card Number 74—29137

Printed in Great Britain

Computer Typesetting by Print Origination, Bootle, Merseyside, L20 6NS

PREFACE

Many ophthalmic texts fail to help those for whom they were primarily written. They are too brief for clarity, and too comprehensive for brevity. Furthermore, they describe all conditions on a system-linked basis, as though they were peculiar to the eye. In fact, many of these maladies are 'ocular' only because of their position.

There are, of course, conditions that are of specialist interest, but all too often they lie hidden behind a cloud of ophthalmic jargon that makes most doctors turn away in despair.

This little book offers a new approach. Firstly, it shows that any clinician is already equipped to deal with a host of 'ocular' problems. Secondly, it outlines a simple guide to the handling of the genuine eye troubles that can be so unnerving, like diplopia, squint, or the red eye.

In this second edition, the reasons why have been extended to meet the needs of medical students and all those who may yet have examiners to face.

The information offered is still symptom-linked and based on what I have found to be the most common problems referred to us at the eye hospital. It avoids the abstruse; it eliminates the irrelevant; it destroys a few myths; but most of all I hope it will bring speedy peace of mind to all those faced with lonely decisions.

My grateful thanks are due to Dr Alistair Adams for his wise suggestions on content and layout, to Mrs Christine McKenzie, who patiently typed the everchanging manuscript, and to Mr Ian Lennox who illustrated the second edition.

H.B.C.

CONTENTS

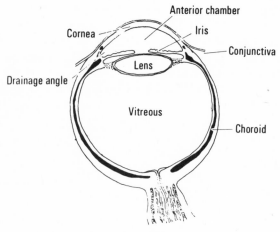

SCHEMATIC CROSS SECTION

Figure 1

SIMPLE EYE DIAGNOSIS
INTRODUCTION

By tradition, most ophthalmic textbooks start with a section on anatomy, then go on to examination methods. Anatomy becomes much clearer when described in relation to various disease processes; thus it will be found scattered throughout the book, wherever relevant.

History taking and examination likewise come more easily to the mind if they are described along with these various diseases.

This section is, therefore, limited to a brief summary of each.

HISTORY TAKING

We have all been well drilled in the art of symptom analysis—routinely probing the duration, mode of onset, associated complaints and so on.

The eye is in no way different. There are only four main themes with variations, and these are amplifed in the various sections:

Visual disturbance
Diplopia
Pain
Discharge and watering (epiphora).

EXAMINATION

The only first-line instrument is a good ophthalmoscope, like the Keeler practitioner. (Fig.2)

Second-line equipment is optional, but at least should include:

> A pinhole disc
> A small magnifying glass
> A wall chart of letters.

The ophthalmoscope

The ophthalmoscope (Fig.2) carries a refraction disc of lenses that neutralize the refractive error of both patient *and* doctor.

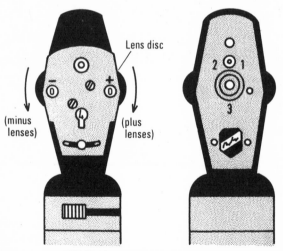

KEELER PRACTITIONER OPHTHALMOSCOPE

Figure 2

Thus if the normal-sighted doctor wants a clear fundal view of a myope he rotates the disc from the zero point anti-clockwise, bringing the black numbered, minus lenses into play. This pushes the focus back onto the distant retina. If the eye is long sighted, clockwise rotation pulls the focus forward.

If the doctor has glasses, he can opt to wear them or discard them. Should he choose to do the latter, he must make up his own refractive error on the disc (this is now his zero point), before attending to the examination and refractive error of the patient.

The ophthalmoscope is a versatile instrument, also serving as a useful light source and as a means of detecting opacities in the cornea, lens and vitreous. Two useful tricks demonstrate this versatility.

The instrument, set at the doctor's zero point, is directed at the patient's eye from about a foot away. Normally, the examined pupil at this distance fills with a red glow—the red reflex, due to light reflected from the choroid through the transparent retina and through the clear media. (Fig. 3)

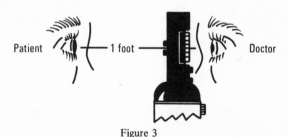

Figure 3

Any opacities in the media show up against this red reflex, and their position can be determined by a further useful manoeuvre: when the ophthalmoscope (and the doctor) move slightly from side to side, the opacities move by parallax. Opacities in the cornea move against the light; in the lens they move not at all, in the vitreous they move with the light. (Fig. 4)

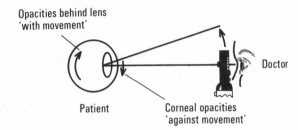

Figure 4

The cornea will come into clear view if the disc is rotated nine notches clockwise from the zero point and if the usual close position for ophthalmoscopy is adopted. The view can then be pushed back through the lens and vitreous by rotating the disc anticlockwise until the retinal detail is in focus.

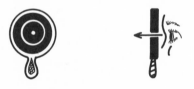

PINHOLE DISC

Figure 5

The pinhole disc

This pocket-sized disc, costing next to nothing, can substitute for a whole box of trial lenses. (Fig. 5)

The principle is that of the pinhole camera. Peripheral light rays are excluded and only axial rays are allowed to pass. All refractive errors are thus nullified. Many people with refractive errors subconsciously come as near to this as nature will allow, by narrowing their eyelid aperture to a slit, thus improving their visual acuity and delaying the cost of a pair of spectacles.

The test with the pinhole disc

With one eye covered, the patient views the letter chart at 6 metres distance, through the pinhole; should the vision improve, then any previous visual loss may be ascribed to an uncorrected error of refraction.

Since visual loss gives rise to a large number of outpatient referrals, it is clear that the pinhole disc goes a long way towards separating the simple spectacle problems from the rest.

The small magnifying lens

This lens works simply by allowing a closer look at the eye than would otherwise be possible. Even without the lens, a good deal of ocular pathology would be recognized if only doctors would shorten their examination distance. This cannot be stressed enough; detail cannot be discerned from afar in any situation.

In a way, the lens forces this close habit on the doctor, because of its short focal distance. Illumination can come from the ophthalmoscopic main beam. If this beam is manoeuvered slowly, from the front to side positions, then all manner of unsuspected diagnoses may appear as well as the beauties of the fine ocular structure.

Wall charts

These will be found, as a rule, in fixed situations like surgeries and ward side-rooms. Those familiar, faded, yellow heirlooms should be discarded in favour of something whiter, and the test distance should be 6 metres. With a bright chart and good lighting, normal distance vision is taken as 6/6. The upper 6 is the test distance in metres. The lower 6 tells the distance at which the patient ought to be able to see the letter size. Thus 6/12 means that the patient can see only at 6 metres what the normal eye could see at 12 metres . . . and so on. If the vision is less than 6/12, then a number plate at 25 yards would be a blur; so might an oncoming vehicle.

Distance vision is not the whole story. Some refractive errors never correct up to a good distance acuity (e.g. severe astigmatism). However, if small reading print can be made out, then the central retina can be taken as normal.

NORMAL VISION

Vision means different things to different people, and the first step towards understanding patients with visual complaints is to realize that vision of each eye has two basic components, central vision and field of vision.

CENTRAL VISION

The tiny retinal area lateral to the optic disc is called the macula. This is highly developed and is stimulated when the eye fixes visually, e.g. looking at a car number-plate. (Fig. 6)

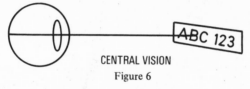

CENTRAL VISION

Figure 6

FIELD OF VISION

The remaining retina makes the eye aware of the surrounding world, which might include another car. (Fig. 7)

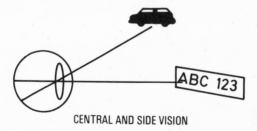

CENTRAL AND SIDE VISION

Figure 7

Central vision further splits into:
    Distance vision
    Near vision (e.g. reading).

DISTANCE VISION

The normal eye
    Relaxed focus at infinity. (Fig. 8)

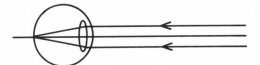

The normal-sighted eye—
relaxed at infinity, i.e. at any
point beyond 6 metres

Figure 8

Short sight (myopia)
    The relaxed focus is well short of infinity; beyond point F (Fig. 9) all is blurred and cannot be seen without a concave (minus lens) which will push point F to infinity.

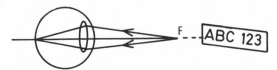

The short-sighted eye—
relaxed short of infinity

Figure 9

Long sight (hypermetropia)
    This eye can never focus in the relaxed state (Fig. 10). A convex lens (plus) with more focusing power will pull the

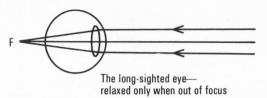

The long-sighted eye—
relaxed only when out of focus

Figure 10

focus (F) up to the retina. Alternatively, the eye can alter the convexity of its own lens by accommodation—in other words, by using its ciliary muscle to increase its focusing power.

Astigmatism

Optically, the astigmatic eye is not a perfect sphere, having different refractive errors in different meridians. Any lens has to correct each meridian separately; in practice, this is achieved usually with a cylindrical lens which produces a focus in one meridian only.

NEAR VISION

The normal eye has to increase the convexity of its own lens to read or to maintain any near focus. (Fig. 11)

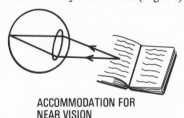

ACCOMMODATION FOR
NEAR VISION
Figure 11

The myopic eye is focused for near anyway.

The hypermetropic eye may have to make enormous demands on its ciliary muscle to maintain a near focus, and may need help, even in youth.

After the age of 40, the lens hardens and increasingly resists the muscle's attempts to give more focusing power.

Thus all people after this age need stronger and stronger reading additions to their own distance prescriptions as the years roll on.

Finally, the visual pathway runs from the retina to the occipital cortex. (Fig. 12)

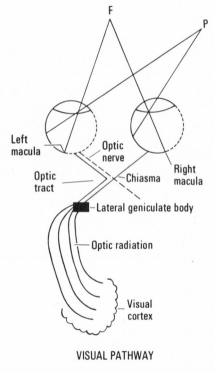

VISUAL PATHWAY

Figure 12

Beyond the chiasma, the left optic tract and radiation transmit impulses from corresponding points in the left half of the retina and the left half of the right retina. These impulses give spatial information about the right visual field (point P). The macular areas overlap on the right and left halves of each retina and are seen fixing on point F.

VISUAL COMPLAINTS AND
METHODS OF EXAMINATION

When patients say they cannot see, an amalgam of ignorance and fear stops them from saying exactly how. A clear history, as ever, is critical and may often give the diagnosis. The following questions should be asked as a matter of course.

Is the visual loss total or partial?
Which eye, or both?
Does the side vision seem normal?
Was the loss sudden or gradual?

EXAMINATION

The routine should be the unchanging tetrad of:

Visual acuity (one eye at a time)
Pupil reaction
Hand movement field
Fundal examination (with the pupil dilated).

Visual acuity

If no test type is available, fixing on any distant object will do. A popular one is the television screen, and there is certain to be one around.

Grading of vision would then be:

Normal
Impaired
Grossly impaired (finger counting)
No perception of light, or bare hand-movement seen only.

Pupil reaction

The pupil reactions are dealt with elswhere (Fig. 21).

Hand movement field

The hand movement or confrontation field is part of the routine cranial nerve assessment. Each eye must be tested separately—with the other covered.

Fundal examination

It is futile to comment on a fundus unless the pupil is dilated, yet house physicians are daily expected to unravel its mysteries, with a waning ophthalmoscope, in a sunlit ward and no mention is made of dilating the pupil. This may be because no suitable dilating agent is to hand. Homatropine is traditional, but Mydrilate (cyclopentolate) is preferable because of its short action.

However short their action may be, these drugs should not be used if *angle closure glaucoma* is suspected (figs. 23, 27, 28.)

PAINLESS LOSS OF VISION
UNILATERAL

Sudden total loss

This is usually due to occlusion of the central retinal artery or of the arterioles in the optic nerve or optic nerve head and is found in the older age groups.

EXAMINATION

Visual acuity—no light perception.

The pupil shows loss of direct reflex on the affected side (inflow defect).

The disc may be swollen.

The retina may be creamy white except for the cherry spot at the macula.

A combination of hypertension and arteriolosclerosis may usually be implicated, but temporal arteritis must be assumed in the over sixties until disproved.

ACTION

Systemic steroids should be started—40 mg of prednisolone daily, until a low erythrocyte sedimentation rate (ESR) has ruled out temporal arteritis.

If the ESR is above 45 mm in the first hour, then a temporal artery biopsy should be carried out at the nearest eye hospital.

Most patients give inaccurate histories and may complain of visual loss in one eye when they, in fact, mean the field on that side. This will be discussed under 'Bilateral visual loss'.

Sudden partial loss

Five likely causes spring to mind:

Occlusion of the central retinal vein or a branch of it

Optic neuritis

Retinal detachment

Vitreous haemorrhage

Sudden awareness of longstanding poor vision.

Central venous occlusion (older age groups)

Visual acuity is usually down to finger counting.

The hand movement field shows some distortion.

The fundal picture is that of the 'stormy sunset' retina, where the turmoil of flame haemorrhages and swollen veins is unforgettable.

If a branch vein is occluded, the field loss will be negligible, and the 'stormy sunset' localized usually to the vein which runs from the disc above the macula. (Fig. 13)

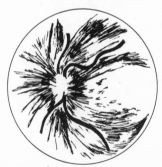

CENTRAL RETINAL VEIN OCCLUSION (LEFT)
Figure 13

ACTION

Diabetes and hypertension should be excluded.

The patient should be referred to an eye hospital, since the occlusion may be a forewarning of chronic glaucoma.

Optic neuritis (younger age group)

Visual acuity may be down beyond finger counting to hand movements, or less.

The pupil shows a sluggish direct reflex on the affected side (inflow defect).

The hand movement field may show good side vision.

The disc may be swollen (optic neuritis—Fig. 19) or normal (retrobulbar neuritis).

ACTION

Reassurance that the vision will return almost to its original level can be given.

It is not necessary to tell the patient that there is a 50 per cent chance of multiple sclerosis developing sometime.

Some authorities use systemic steroids, other authorities, of equal standing, do not.

Referral to an eye clinic, sometime, will at least give some comfort to the patient, while the vision improves without treatment.

Retinal detachment (any age group, but most frequently in myopia or following cataract extraction)

Visual acuity may be normal or anything down to light perception if the central area is involved.

Hand movement field loss will correspond to the area of detachment.

A grey, rippling appearance will take the place of the normal red reflex. (Fig. 14)

ACTION

This is an emergency and should be referred to an eye department, at once.

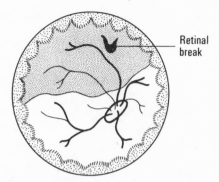

RIGHT RETINAL DETACHMENT (UPPER TEMPORAL)

Figure 14

Vitreous haemorrhage (any age group)
Visual acuity may be reduced to light perception only.
A black reflex will obscure the normal red reflex.

ACTION
Diabetes, hypertension and the 'bleeding diseases' should be tested for.
Referral to an eye clinic sometime soon is indicated.

Sudden awareness of longstanding poor vision
This is discussed in 'The reason why'.

BILATERAL

Sudden partial loss
As already suggested, the real problem is a homonymous field defect (Fig. 12) appearing to the patient as sudden total visual loss in one eye.
Visual acuity may be normal.
Hand movement field testing will show an equal defect to the same side of the fixation point in each eye.

The cause is usually a vascular accident behind the midbrain so the pupil reflexes will be normal.

ACTION

Hypertension, diabetes and blood disorders should be excluded.

Sources of embolus must be sought.

Referral to an eye department will help to determine the treatable causes in the hope of preventing a similar disaster in the other field.

UNILATERAL

Gradual general loss
>   Choroiditis
>   Creeping inferior retinal detachment
>   Choroidal melanoma.

Choroiditis (may be bilateral at any age, but usually in the young)

Non-specific inflammatory change in the choroid may produce a hazy vitreous with resultant hazy vision.

Visual acuity may be almost normal.

Vitreal haze will be seen with the ophthalmoscope, and the red reflex correspondingly dulled.

ACTION

Rapid referral to an eye clinic is imperative, where the prescription of systemic steroids may prevent severe ocular damage.

Creeping inferior retinal detachment (may be bilateral and usually the younger age group)

The cause is often a congenital weakness in the peripheral retina or a long forgotten injury. It may only be noticed when the lifting retina catches the macula thus reducing central vision.

Visual acuity will vary with the mode of presentation (i.e. whether it presents as a field defect or as central visual loss).

A flat, grey reflex will replace the red reflex in the lower fundus.

Similar earlier changes may be found in the other eye.

ACTION
Referral for detachment surgery sometime soon is indicated.

Choroidal melanoma (usually in the over forties)
The presentation resembles that of a creeping retinal detachment.

Fundal examination may reveal anything from a mottled grey/black shallow detachment to a round, solid dark lump of varying size.

ACTION
Referral for specialist care is advised although not necessarily as an emergency.

Enucleation is the standard approach, although sometimes, a small tumour, uncomplicated by a secondary retinal detachment may be excised. Routine chest X-ray in all cases will screen the favourite site for metastatic deposits.

BILATERAL

Gradual general loss
        Senile cataract
        Chronic glaucoma
        Diabetic retinopathy
        Hypertensive retinopathy
        Pituitary adenoma.

Senile cataract

Visual acuity may be anything down to light perception.

The fundal view is made hazy by a grey reflex in the pupil (Fig. 3). However, this need not prevent ophthalmoscopy through the dilated pupil.

ACTION

If the fundus looks normal, and the patient is seeing to get around, then surgery need not be hurried into.

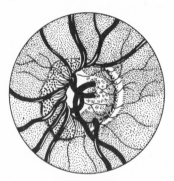

CUPPED DISC

Figure 15

Chronic glaucoma (older age groups)

This condition is common and sinister—sinister because it is usually symptomless until it has damaged the vision grievously.

Visual acuity is usually normal until the late stages.

Hand-movement field testing will show variable loss especially on the nasal side.

The discs will show enlargement of the central cup. (Fig. 15)

ACTION

Specialist care is obligatory for permanent follow-up.

Senile macular degeneration

Visual acuity falls in one or both eyes

Hand movement fields are usually full

The discs are usually normal.

The macular changes range from a fine pigmentary stipple to raised fibrous scars or frank haemorrhage.

Diabetic retinopathy

Duration rather than severity of diabetes is the keynote in the development of this condition.

In this context, the central macular exudates are to blame.

ACTION

This is fully discussed as a separate section.

Hypertensive retinopathy

As with diabetes, the relevent aspect here is macular affection, either oedema, exudate or haemorrhage.

ACTION

This is fully discussed as a separate section.

Pituitary adenoma

The enlarging pituitary gland causes a variety of conditions, but if it compresses the optic chiasma, irregular visual damage will ensue.

Visual acuity may be normal, but with a vague hint of subnormality.

Hand-movement field changes, classically bitemporal but more often irregular, are found.

Perhaps a more arresting feature is the well-known but often ignored facies of pituitary deficiency.

The discs may show pallor due to longstanding compression.

ACTION

A full ophthalmic, endocrine and neurosurgical examination is the necessary prelude to neurosurgery.

THE REASON WHY

The foregoing list does not attempt to be complete, but it touches on aspects of ophthalmology that may have caused recurrent confusion in the past. For instance, many students and elderly doctors pursue their careers unaware that optic neuritis and retrobulbar neuritis are, in fact, the same condition, which strikes different parts of the optic nerve. The former is visible as a swollen disc (Fig. 19), and the latter hides its swelling further back in the nerve and the diagnosis is made by inference and exclusion.

Retinal detachment

Simple retinal detachment must always be due to retinal tears and a degenerate vitreous. The large myopic eye has not enough retina to go round, thus tears develop more readily at the equator which is about as far out as the direct ophthalmoscope can reach. Retinae following cataract extraction develop tears even further out. If the vitreous becomes more fluid than normal, then it will flow through these tears, peeling the neural retina away from its pigment layer. Cut off from half its blood supply, the retina starves, and early surgery (within a few days) is preferred.

However, as long as there is perception of light, it is never too late, and in the hands of a retinal specialist the operative success rate should be over 90 per cent.

It is worth noting that tumours, inflammation and diabetic traction bands can all cause secondary retinal detachment.

The sine qua non of surgery is to find and seal the retinal break. A temporary seal can be achieved by buckling the ocular layers inwards with silicone rubber or sponge stitched on to the sclera.

Floating the retinal break on an intra-vitreal air bubble is a much gentler way of doing the same thing.

The permanent seal is produced by prior application of some inflammatory agent—like diathermy or nowadays cryo-coagulation—which forms a watertight chorio-retinal scar, over the same period of time required for any inflammatory process to end in scar tissue.

Apparent visual loss

Sudden awareness of long standing poor vision is commoner than might be expected. People who might offer an informed view on a galaxy of subjects can be remarkably unaware of their own visual standards. Rather than assume ignorance and miss some dangerous neurological cause, it is better to refer these cases for a specialist's opinion, should any reasonable doubt remain.

Cataract

The bulk of referrals to eye clinics must be due to cataract. Now, technically, any lens opacity is called a cataract, but it is a name that often evokes an image of blindness and a deal of terror. The most tragic proof of this fear came from a man, almost irretrievably blind from untreated glaucoma, who remarked, 'Thank goodness, it is not cataract!' His relief was ill-founded.

Sometimes a cataract becomes very ripe and soft, when it should be removed before it bursts into the eye and causes a fiery inflammation. At all other times, the indication for surgery is the patient's failure to function in his own environment. Vision following extraction, corrected with suitable thick glasses is very different from normal vision, in that objects directly viewed are magnified and the field of vision diminished. Thus an eye in this situation cannot balance optically with its normal fellow with simple glasses. A contact lens, substituting for the removed lens, is the nearest simple approach to a normal balance. There has, however, been a vogue for placing an acrylic lens inside the eye—a procedure not without its complications and hence not widely practised.

Glaucoma

Now, while early cataract needing no treatment will produce a stream of anxious patients, glaucoma too advanced for effective control may be almost without symptoms at all.

Although not strictly accurate semantically, glaucoma is now taken to mean an elevation of the ocular pressure above 'normal'. Anything that blocks the flow of aqueous, either through the pupil (e.g. ring adhesions from iritis) or out of the eye, will give rise to glaucoma. Narrow-angle glaucoma is discussed elsewhere, and all manner of conditions from the pathology list of trauma, neoplasia, etc. can result in secondary glaucoma.

The sinister glaucoma is where, for some unknown reason, aqueous drainage from the eye begins to fail. The whole eye has a more faltering blood supply, and the optic nerve capillaries succumb more quickly to a pressure that might not affect a healthy young eye. The rising pressure squeezes the visual field out of existence, but leaves central vision intact to the end. This explains the late presentation for treatment; it also explains the behaviour of the elderly, who cannot understand why they are being subjected to regular examination, regular drop medication or to major eye surgery.

Regular examination at a glaucoma clinic allows the doctor to check the efficacy of treatment which generally involves the following drugs

G.pilocarpine, increases the outflow of aqueous through the anterior chamber angle (Fig. 27)

G.Eppy (stable adrenaline) reduces the aqueous at its source as well as increasing its outflow from the eye.

Acetazolamide by mouth can be used even on its own to cut down the formation of aqueous.

All these, therefore, reduce the intra-ocular pressure.

If field loss and disc cupping continue, despite maximal medication, then the surgeon must try to fashion a drainage channel from the anterior chamber to the subconjunctival space. This surgery unhappily may do little to stabilise the glaucoma, however it will usually manage to increase existing lens opacities or to produce them where there were none before. Even so, progressive loss of vision frequently leaves us with no choice.

Most chronic glaucoma is picked up at routine examination for something else. The message here must be that all people over 40 require a regular eye check at a medical eye centre or at an optician's every two years, no matter how good their present glasses are.

Senile macular degeneration

This behaves, visually, as the reverse of glaucoma, in that the central vision gradually fails, but the visual field stays intact.

The capillary blood supply to the macula breaks down. The macular part of the retinal pigment layer and the layer deep to that (Bruch's membrane) both atrophy—hence the patchy depigmentation and the rupture of choroidal vessels through into the retina.

Although some degenerations might be treatable with laser therapy, most progress mercilessly until even a hand-magnifier does nothing for the reading capacity. Fortunately, it is possible to reassure these worried old folk that they are not going to 'go blind'; they will keep their side vision despite the failure of their reading vision.

Pituitary Adenoma

Because of anatomical variations, visual field defects alone can only suggest the likely diagnosis.

Metabolic studies for pituitary dysfunction will help confirm the clinical findings. However, before the head is opened, the neuroradiologist must do both air studies to demonstrate any possible supra-sellar extension and angiograms to exclude the possibility of an intra-cranial aneurysm.

Tobacco Amblyopia

Addicts of black Cavendish, especially those who flavour their addiction with hard spirits, may over the years begin to lose their central vision. Failing red/green discrimination and eventual optic atrophy only confirm a suspicion that the history should have already raised.

Cyanide from powerful tobacco overwhelms the enzyme systems that in normal circumstances would have turned it into harmless thiocyanate. This pitiless decline of macular function can be halted by parenteral hydroxocobalamin 1000 μg twice weekly.

To sum up, it is worth mentioning the value of the pinhole disc for separating refractive errors from genuine pathology. Thereafter, approaching the various riddles according to the simple system outlined in the previous section must remove much of the terror from these conditions for the doctor at least. Perhaps we can remember this method best by para-phrasing an old military maxim into a medical one, 'Divide and diagnose.'

VAGUE VISUAL SYMPTOMS

Fleeting visual loss

This subject is complex, involving possibly the heart, the great vessels to the head, or the cerebral arteries. Anaemia, embolic episodes from any source, hypertension or hypotension can all play their part in distressing the patient.

The patterns of migraine and postural hypotension are well known, and can be diagnosed on their history alone. However, as can be seen from this grim catalogue, a formidable group remains whose symptoms call for a practised and thorough investigation. The embolic episodes, especially, may be the forerunners of more tragic and more permanent visual impairment in the not distant future.

ACTION

These symptoms must be regarded as urgent.

Floaters

Simple

These are the so-called muscae volitantes, fine wisps and tendrils that float with the eye movements and show up most strikingly against a white background or sunlit sky.

Fine vitreous opacities are to blame, flinging their shadow on the retina and often causing much distress.

ACTION

Reassurance.

Complicated

When other symptoms join with the floaters, they may be heralds of serious ocular disease. Sudden floaters with impaired vision may follow, vitreous haemorrhage—itself often due to diabetes, hypertension, or a retinal tear.

Retinal detachment   This may, on its own, cause a vitreous haemorrhage which, of course, obscures the underlying detachment. The onset of flashing lights in this situation usually means a retinal tear which may lead on to a detachment.

Iritis Although usually presenting as a red eye, iritis occasionally scatters inflammatory debris across the visual line in the anterior chamber.

Choroiditis This is fully explained later on but it behaves like iritis in all but position.

ACTION

A routine urinary glucose and protein test and blood pressure check should be followed by referral to hospital.

Haloes

Angle-closure glaucoma classically gives early warning of its presence in this way. Fading daylight dilates the pupil and produces a partial angle block that elevates the intraocular pressure. Consequent upon this, a dull ache settles above the eyebrow, and the water-logged cornea splits light into rainbow rings with incidental visual blurring (Fig. 23).

ACTION

Pilocarpine 2 per cent will unblock the angle by constricting the pupil. This will serve until the patient can be seen at an eye clinic. An additional safety measure would be Diamox 500 mg stat by mouth, but in the absence of a full-blown attack of acute glaucoma this is not strictly necessary.

Flashing lights

This common sensation implies irritation of some kind or other in either the retina or the visual cortex. Both these highly refined tissues can give only the impression of light flashing. Stimulate them as we will, that will be their response. Seeing stars, following a blow to the head, must be familiar to all devotees of cartoons and comic strips; perhaps the explanation is less familiar.

Since elimination of needless investigations is almost as important as a correct diagnosis, we must segregate the significant from the casual, and a good history will do just this.

Retinal lesions

The complaint will be of persistent, unilateral localized light flashes. These cease abruptly after some days or weeks in a fine shower of visual floaters.

The patient is, in fact, describing the formation of a retinal break. The vitreous, abnormally adherent in one area, begins to tug on the light-sensitive retina, hence the flashes, giving way to a shower of floaters which may be of pigment or of frank blood.

ACTION

Fairly rapid referral to an eye clinic where a freeze-induced or light induced inflammatory barrier around the tear may prevent a full-blown retinal detachment.

Odd light flashes may persist after retinal surgery, but of

course there has then been enough ocular manipulation to account for them.

Other lesions

Usually due to disturbance in the cerebral blood flow, these give rise to vague, swooping light-streaking with no distinctive pattern. Migraine or the foretokens of a tumour will usually attract the attention of both patient and physician with features more striking than mere light flashes.

ACTION

If the cranial nerves and blood pressure are normal, then the doctor must rely on his 'nose' for the serious when assessing these common symptoms.

THE NORMAL DISC AND SOME
ABNORMAL DISC SYDNROMES

The normal disc

The normal optic disc (Fig. 16) presents to the observer

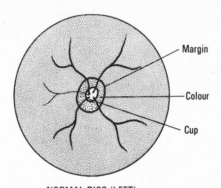

NORMAL DISC (LEFT)

Figure 16

three main features, coming readily to the mind with the letters MCC:

M—margin which should be sharp but may be blurred in extreme long sight.

C—colour, varying from pale (short sight) to dark red (long sight).

C—cup, central and physiological that should be no greater than one-quarter the disc size. In long sight it may be minute. There may be a cresecent on the temporal or inferior margins where the absent pigment epithelium exposes the white sclera.(Fig. 17)

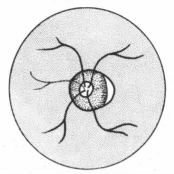

MYOPIC DISC WITH TEMPORAL CRESCENT (LEFT)

Figure 17

The apparently swollen disc

Pseudo-papilloedema, where the disc appears swollen, but in fact is not; the vessels are not engorged, and only the disc margins are actually blurred. It is perhaps more common in extreme cases of long sight. (Fig. 18)

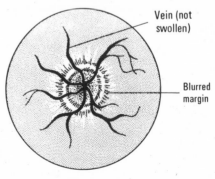

Vein (not swollen)

Blurred margin

PSEUDO-PAPILLOEDEMA (LEFT)

Figure 18

ACTION

When there is any doubt, a full ophthalmic assessment is needed to decide if the disc is in fact swollen, and if so why?

When the disc is really swollen,

M—the margin is blurred;

C—the colour is very red; also dilated veins, haemorrhages and extension of oedema on to adjacent retina;

C—the cup is diminished. (Fig. 19)

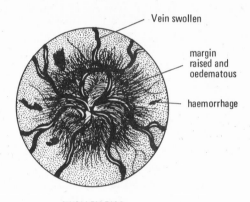

Vein swollen

margin
raised and
oedematous

haemorrhage

SWOLLEN DISC
Figure 19

The retinal veins and the surrounding retina join in the general engorgement and streaky retinal haemorrhages may be found as well.

Some swollen disc sydromes:
Unilateral

1. Sudden marked *central* visual loss. The most likely cause is optic neuritis (papillitis).

2. Sudden marked visual loss both *central* and *peripheral*. Distended, irregular veins coil and twist through retinal

oedema and flame haemorrhages. Aptly named the 'stormy sunset' fundus, it is due to occlusion of the central retinal vein. (Fig. 13)

Both conditions are discussed under 'Painless visual loss'

Bilateral

With or without mild visual disturbance. This is either (1) malignant hypertension, a diagnosis confirmed by a rocketing blood pressure and soft exudates—or (2) plerocephalic oedema (papilloedema) classically associated with raised intracranial pressure.

ACTION

Referral to an ophthalmic unit is in order.

If the diagnosis is certain and linked with other symptoms and signs of a cerebral tumour, then it is as well to refer straight to a neurologist. If the diagnosis is uncertain, the ophthalmologist can distinguish the genuinely swollen from the apparently swollen disc, by the intravenous injection of sodium fluorescein which leaks from the engorged capillaries of the diseased optic nerve head and lingers in the eye longer than it should.

SQUINT AND DIPLOPIA

Most medical people faced with the complaint of double vision in the adult have a faint recollection of attempts to determine the palsied muscle from the position of the false image. Even fainter is their recollection of just how to manage this palsy once it has been given a name. Squint in the child causes still more bemusement, with fleeting memories of steel-rimmed spectacles, patched eyes and lazy vision.

The apparent complexity leads to prejudice, and prejudice leads to half diagnosis or to no diagnosis at all. The irony is that with a handful of easy facts the difficulties just melt away. Discussing the subject from infancy onwards makes these facts even easier still.

Childhood squints

The eyes are moved collectively by 12 muscles, and if left without any higher control, either eye could point in any direction it chooses.

The brain locks both eyes together so that both central areas join to look at one fixation point at any given time. This is called 'binocular vision' (Fig. 12), and gives us our depth perception and three dimensional sense.

A child born without binocular vision will usually use one eye, letting the other eye wander at will. Rather than tolerate two pictures of the world, he will suppress the wandering one.

If this suppression is not checked before the age of 5 years, the wandering eye will become lazy—physically normal, but with poor central vision. Some authorities would extend this deadline to 8 years, but no-one can dispute that the longer treatment is delayed the less hope there is for visual improvement.

Central vision is a fragile talent before the age of 5 years, and many factors can arrest its development. The earlier this arrest happens, the deeper will be the central visual loss. Anything that blocks a direct approach of light to the central area can do this, e.g. a dropped lid, a corneal scar, a congenital cataract, congenital nystagmus, constantly agitating the central area. Any doctor knows enough pathology to extend this list at will.

In childhood squints
    the eye can move freely and fully;
    there is no muscle palsy;
    the fault lies in the brain and can be thought of as defective binocular vision.

EXAMINATION

The only useful test is to watch the child in the full-face position, then to check the eye movements. The doctor must try to hold the child's interest, and hence his eyes, with some attractive bauble. (We use a little flat stick with a bird at one end and a policeman at the other, to make the child focus.) With luck, the squint will show up. From there, it is an easy step to assess the eye movements and this is, of course, a part of the standard cranial nerve examination.

The important movements are upwards, downwards, and to either side, each eye being tested separately. There are other movements and other manoeuvres, e.g. the cover test, usually given several pages in the textbooks. These tests are for ophthalmologists; on their own they can be misleading, used infrequently they can be dangerous. They should be avoided.

ACTION

Before 5 years of age If a squint is suspected, and a family history may strengthen this, the child should be referred to an eye clinic. We would rather see children with normal eyes, but suspected of squinting, than miss children with abnormal eyes, unsuspected of squinting.

A child will *not* grow out of a squint. The price he pays is the central vision of one eye.

After 5 years of age The problem is becoming solely cosmetic. If the child has not been checked for glasses, this should be done at an optician's or a medical eye centre. Either eye, if lazy, is now beyond improvement.

If the appearance is poor, then cosmetic squint surgery is indicated with no upper age limit.

Adult squint and double vision:

Squints developing in adults generally differ from those of children in two important ways:

the main symptom is double vision,

the main sign is a muscle palsy (*eye movements are not full*).

A further refinement is that the double vision is worse when the weak muscle is in action. However, patients often say 'double vision' when they mean 'blurred vision', and this confusion can be cleared up by direct questioning.

The following sparse details are a prerequisite of clear diagnosis.

Three cranial nerves supply the eye muscles. In reverse order, they are:

the sixth nerve, moving the eye outwards;

the fourth nerve, moving the eye downwards and inwards;

the third nerve moving the eye in all other directions,

and

elevating the upper lid

and

constricting the pupil.

Thus in the affected eye:

a sixth nerve palsy will limit outward movement;

a fourth nerve palsy (rare) will limit downward, inward movement;

a third nerve palsy will limit all other movements

and

will cause a dropped lid

and

a dilated pupil.

These are the only ophthalmic facts necessary. The rest should be common knowledge.

Anatomy

All three nerves start in the brain stem and proceed to the orbit, passing the cavernous sinus and the internal carotid artery on the way (Fig. 20)

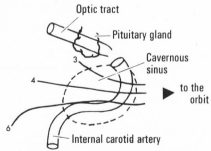

THIRD, FOURTH AND SIXTH CRANIAL NERVES
EN ROUTE TO THE ORBIT

Figure 20

Pathology

The most likely causes are as follows:

Minor vascular lesion in the brain stem (older age groups)

The 'Bell's type' palsy of the sixth nerve (younger age group)

Diabetes

Multiple sclerosis

Myasthenia gravis.

EXAMINATION

With the preceding conditions in mind, the doctor must test: the eye movements; the remaining cranial nerves; the blood pressure; the urine for sugar and protein.

ACTION

Third-nerve malfunctions may connote something ominous, e.g. a cerebral aneurysm, requiring urgent care.

An isolated fourth-nerve palsy almost always results from an obvious injury.

Sixth-nerve weakness is often an isolated event, clearing up totally in about three months. More rarely, it may foreshadow raised intracranial pressure. If this were so, other aspects might raise suspicions, e.g. vague headaches or swelling optic nerve heads (Fig. 19)

In cases of myasthenia gravis, intravenous injection of Tensilon (edrophonium chloride) should transiently eliminate the paralysis.

Latent squint

The most full-proof systems have at least one exception. What if there is a blend of occasional double vision *and* full eye movements? The answer is simple: the central visual axes want to point in different directions and the normal binocular vision fails to hold them together, especially in stressful situations. This is called latent squint and the direction is usually horizontal.

ACTION

Orthoptic care in the first instance may not be enough, and operation could then bring the visual axes nearer to each other.

THE REASON WHY

Any remaining loose strands can now be tied up less briefly.

Spectacles

Long sight (Fig. 10) is a frequent associate of convergent squint because the brain centres for accommodation and convergence are closely linked. When the normal-sighted child or adult focuses to read (Fig. 11), the eyes converge to maintain single vision. The child with uncorrected long sight has to overfocus for near and so has to overconverge as well. In this situation, the role of correcting glasses must now be clear.

Patching

Ideally, the orthoptist aims at perfect binocular vision. In practice, she settles for less, striving for equal vision alternating from one eye to the other. By patching the 'good eye', she persuades the 'lazy' one to work and she strengthens this persuasion with little games designed to interest the lazy macula. The real burden of all this, however, falls on the mother, who will have to blend threats, bribery and cajolery to keep the patch in place during the waking hours. Half-hearted patching is worthless; unsupervised patching may induce amblyopia in the 'good' eye.

Surgery

Operations for squint are generally for cosmetic reasons, but just occasionally they may be used to bring the eyes in line with each other, closely enough to allow the binocular impulses to hold them there (latent squint).

Popular techniques strengthen or weaken the muscles of the squinting eye. However, it is best to think of surgery as seeking to restore balance between the 12 eye muscles, since it is sometimes necessary to operate on the 'good eye'. Fashions vary from centre to centre.

As soon as the angle of squint can be measured (roughly at 18 months), there is no embargo on surgery on grounds of age. The one proviso is that it is customary to delay six months before treating paralytic squint by surgery in case of a spontaneous recovery.

Perhaps this section might best be summed up with a true story. A woman consulted her practitioner because she feared her two-year-old had a squinting eye. 'Oh, she'll grow out of it,' said her doctor and, pointing to his own divergent eyes, he added, 'Nobody's perfect, you know!'

This child was being condemned to probable amblyopia on her doctor's advice. It is also just possible that her doctor was unaware that he, too, might have made effective use of an ophthalmologist for his own blemish.

THE PUPIL REFLEXES AND
SOME COMMON PUPIL ABNORMALITIES

The reflexes

All reflexes behave in the same two ways:
there is a neuromuscular response to a stimulus;
there are outflow and inflow pathways.

The pupils

The response is constriction only.

The outflow is the third cranial nerve from the midbrain.
The stimulus is twofold:

light (a strong torch must be used);

focusing for near vision (accommodation).

The inflow is twofold:

light—travels by the retina and optic nerve to the midbrain.

accommodation—the pathway is still controversial.

Note Any blinding lesion behind the midbrain, e.g. in the occipital cortex, has no influence on the pupil reflexes. If the left eye is stimulated, *both* pupils will constrict. This would be called the left direct response and the right consensual response (Fig. 21).

The defective light reflexes
Inflow defect

If only the left direct and right consensual reflexes are lost, this means a left inflow defect, e.g. occlusion of the left central retinal artery.

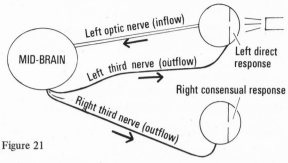

Figure 21

Strong illumination of the normal right eye would in this case, constrict the right and the left pupils. The left consensual response would be present, i.e. the left outflow would be normal.

Outflow defect

If only the left direct and left consensual reflexes are lost, this means a left outflow defect, e.g. third nerve palsy. In this case, the right direct and right consensual reflexes would be present.

ACTION

This must include:
a brisk survey of the cranial nerves;
a blood-pressure reading;
tests for urinary glucose and protein;
blood test for syphilis.

None of these procedures includes any manoeuvre that is not already second nature to all clinicians.

Common pupil abnormalities

Unequal, but with normal light reactions

This may be normal, a conviction confirmed by a negative examination.

Unilateral

Dilated, with a sluggish or absent light reflex (direct and consensual)

This is the Holmes Adie pupil which by tradition is linked with absent jerk reflexes, but in practice, much more likely to be associated with a failure of near focus. If the eye can still focus for near, the pupil will constrict (accommodation reflex). The constriction and subsequent dilatation will be remarkably slow.

ACTION

Reassurance—following the examination routine.

Dilated and fixed

Inadvertent instillation of a mydriatic, e.g. atropine, is commoner than might be imagined.

Following a history of trauma; this in itself is not dangerous, but it must be remembered that a blow severe enough to paralyse the sphincter may have caused other damage.

In serious conditions, like acute glaucoma or a third-nerve palsy, the dilated pupil is often picked up as an incidental finding amongst other more florid presenting features.

Small with abnormal direct light reflex

Horner's syndrome is due to some affection of the cervical sympathetic running from the spinal cord to the brain via the carotid arteries. There is an associated ptosis, if it is remembered that fear, mediated by the sympathetic, can dilate the pupil, then the small pupil of sympathetic paralysis can be easily worked out.

ACTION

This should be on general principles. Horner's syndrome in itself is rare, but, if found, it more often than not points to some mass at the thoracic outlet.

Small and fixed

Instillation of miotic drops, e.g. pilocarpine.

The Argyll-Robertson pupil is often confused with the Holmes-Adie pupil. A refined point is that although the light reflex is gone, the accommodation reflex is not. It has been likened to a student's garret of olden times, as having 'accommodation, but no light'. With venereal diseases again on the rampage, the ability to recognise the luetic pupil is surely an invaluable talent.

ACTION

It is probably wiser to presume the patient to be infective until a venereal expert has given an opinion.

Although pontine haemorrhage and narcotic poisoning are customarily described with pinpoint pupils, these latter would only add weight to a collection of more striking neurological proofs.

Now, not all abnormal pupils have abnormal reflexes. Local conditions can alter the regular round appearance even though the reflex pathways are still intact.

Injury, either accidental or surgical, can leave gaps in the iris running from the pupil margin to the iris root.

A rarer, though physically similar, defect is the developmental coloboma. (Fig. 22)

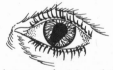

IRIS COLOBOMA
(LEFT)
Figure 22

Adhesions between the iris and the lens frequently follow iritis. If all the way round the pupil margin, they may block the aqueous flow from the ciliary body to the anterior chamber with a resultant secondary glaucoma.

In all these situations, a bright torch will still elicit some remnant of the normal reflex responses.

THE RED EYE

Traditionally, the red eye is presented as a table with multiple causes set against multiple signs; in fact, one drug company has brought out a slide rule for ease of diagnosis with the appropriate brand therapy, slipping in and out with the centre piece.

Although clarity is the aim, the mind recoils from such a diagnostic jumble and may take refuge in the dangerous, catch-all combinations of antibiotics and steroids.

A simpler approach is to divide up the patient's complaints as follows.

Eyes that are PAINFUL and also happen to be red   This group includes:
> Acute glaucoma
> Acute iritis
> Corneal afflictions (foreign bodies, abrasions, ulcers).

Eyes that are RED and also happen to be painful   This group includes:
> Conjunctivitis
> Episcleritis.
> Spontaneous subconjunctival haemorrhage.

Note   All these conditions can be diagnosed with a strong torch and two basic observations.

The corneal surface

In health, this sparkles and glistens when illuminated. Damage to the corneal surface epithelium can dull the lustre, and an ulcer or an abrasion will produce an actual break in this layer. A deeper break will produce a permanent scar.

The green dye, fluorescein, will outline and stain the defects when they are examined in the torchlight (Fig. 37).

The pupil reflex

In this situation, it is simply the response to the same torchlight; noting its original starting size compared with the fellow pupil is also helpful.

PAINFUL EYES THAT HAPPEN TO BE RED

Acute glaucoma

The cornea is hazy but not staining.

The pupil is half dilated and fixed (Fig. 23).

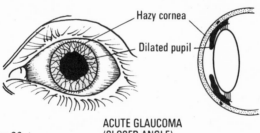

Hazy cornea

Dilated pupil

ACUTE GLAUCOMA
(CLOSED ANGLE)

Figure 23

Both eyes will have a shallow anterior chamber.

The draining angle ('a' in Fig. 27) is blocked by the dilating pupil, and the acute rise of intraocular pressure causes crippling pain.

ACTION

Diamox 500 mg should be given by mouth or by intra-muscular injection, followed by 250 mg 6 hourly, to reduce the intraocular pressure.

Guttae (G.) pilocarpine 2 per cent should be poured into the eye to constrict the pupil and open the angle ('a', Fig. 27).

G. pilocarpine 2 per cent should be instilled about 6 hourly to the fellow eye to avoid a similar catastrophe on that side.

Note   Instant referral to an eye clinic is mandatory. This is a real emergency where delay can cost the vision of both eyes.

Acute iritis

The cornea is clear.

The pupil is spastic (small). (Fig. 24)

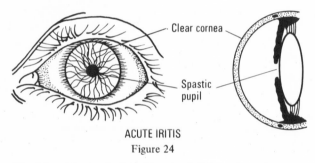

ACUTE IRITIS
Figure 24

The iris sphincter irritated by the inflammation clamps down, causing pain deep in the eye.

ACTION

G. atropine 1 per cent should be instilled 6 hourly to dilate the pupil.

Local steroids should be instilled hourly to reduce the inflammation, but *only* if the cornea is not staining. This latter point cannot be overemphasized.

Referral to an eye department within 24 to 48 hours is called for.

Corneal afflictions

Ulcer or abrasion

The cornea stains with fluorescein (Fig. 37) in the area of defective epithelium.

The pupil may be spastic if there is a secondary iritis.

Corneal foreign body

This will be seen on the corneal surface on *close* examination. It is vital to ascertain from the history if this was travelling fast enough to enter the globe. The eye may be little deranged by this disaster

ACTION

Corneal ulcer

G.atropine 1 per cent should be instilled to dilate the pupil.

Local antibiotic drops should be instilled every 6 hours to avert secondary infection.

A pad stuck down with Sellotape will ease the patient's discomfort.

Superficial corneal foreign bodies

These may be brushed off with a cotton-tipped stick, and perhaps a local anaesthetic drop such as G. amethocaine will make this less trying for patient and physician alike. If this fails, a sterile injection needle will cause less damage than the traditional corneal 'spud' which is about as delicate as its name.

Dendritic ulcers

These are a special case—since they are both common and difficult to treat, and may result in devastating visual loss; they are also recurrent. The *Herpes simplex* virus which causes them is found in cold sores, but may have no obvious source, since it is a commensal in the conjunctiva, hence the frequency of recurrence.

Fluorescein reveals the typical branching figure (Fig. 25).

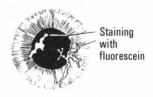

Staining
with
fluorescein

DENDRITIC ULCER
Figure 25

ACTION

In hospital, the freshly staining areas are usually cauterised with an orange stick dipped in phenol or absolute alcohol. Smaller ulcers may respond to gutt. Idoxuridine—a specific antiviral agent. *On no account should steroids be used. In the presence of a dendritic ulcer, their use amounts to malpractice.*

THE RED EYE THAT HAPPENS TO BE PAINFUL

Acute conjunctivitis

The corneal lustre is normal.

The pupil is normal.

Acute conjunctivits is usually bacterial, especially if there is a discharge; but allergy, virus infections and non-specific grumbling inflammations can all cause conjunctivitis.

ACTION

Culture should be taken of any discharge.

Intensive G.chloramphenicol, hourly or more often, should be applied. A pad actually hinders recovery.

Viral conjunctivitis will take its own time, usually about three weeks, but antibiotics will limit secondary infections—a general medical principle.

Episcleritis:

There is an isolated, often raised patch of inflammation.
The corneal lustre is normal. (Fig. 26)
The pupil is normal.

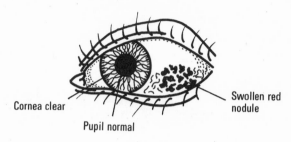

Cornea clear

Pupil normal

Swollen red nodule

EPISCLERITIS

Figure 26

ACTION

If there is no corneal stain, then a short, sharp course of local steroids will quickly clear this up.

Subconjunctival haemorrhage

Like episcleritis the red patch is localized. However the clue to diagnosis lies in the absence of conjunctival vascular markings, obscured by the haemorrhage and the transient dragging ache at the time of onset.

ACTION

The first step should be reassurance to the often frightened patient. Thereafter, one can pursue the general causes of spontaneous haemorrhage on general principles.

THE REASON WHY

Acute glaucoma

This condition is the result of an unfortunate collection of chances. Before it can happen the pupil must dilate. Now the pupil dilates in two circumstances, in the dark (actually the reverse of the light reflex) and when the sympathetic system goes into action; the eyes dilating with fright is a cliché in certain types of literature. But the pupil dilatation is not enough, else everyone would suffer acute glaucoma at dusk. The drainage angle ('a', Fig. 27) must be narrow.

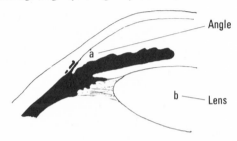

CROSS SECTION SHOWING DRAINAGE ANGLE

Figure 27

Narrow angles are found in small overcrowded eyes, and these are usually long sighted. But young hypermetropes tend not to suffer acute attacks of glaucoma, so some other factor must be added. Effectively, this factor is a forward movement of the lens ('b') as the years go by, and further narrowing may be enough to block the angle in the right situation.

The stage is now set for catastrophe. Transient haloes, blurred vision and pain above the eyebrow give advance warning of this calamity, and if it is heeded, the likelihood may be averted.

The eye at risk can be recognized by its shallow anterior chamber when the forward bowing of the iris eclipses the light, as shown in Fig. 28. The person at risk is usually an edgy, long sighted, middle-aged female. This apparent whimsy is often true. It would he hard to forget a particular woman, who when

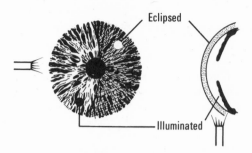

SHALLOW ANTERIOR CHAMBER

Figure 28

told what her 10 years of haloes meant, worried herself into an attack of acute glaucoma in each eye on her way home, *despite constricting drops.*

Acute iritis

Although found in association with some conditions like rheumatoid arthritis, ankylosing spondylitis gonorrhoea, Reiter's urethritis or sarcoidosis, iritis is really a disease on its own.

Inflammatory adhesions and exudative debris can block aqueous flow at two sites. Between the pupil margins and the lens ('b', Fig. 27) and the drainage angle ('a'). If adhesions must form, then G.atropine will ensure their happening in the dilated position. The adhesions then will have a harder time completing the circle of the pupil margin and pupil block glaucoma is less likely. The resultant vision is also better if the debris is at the lens periphery and for obvious reasons.

Irregular iris–lens adhesions that may have developed during previous episodes will sometimes disguise the 'spastic-pupil' sign. Even so, they will not hide the spastic trend wherever a stretch of the pupil sphincter has managed to escape from the restraint of fibrosis.

Keratitis

For all practical purposes, any breach in the corneal epithelium can be described as keratitis. The form of the breach varies with the cause but the uptake of the dye fluorescein (Figs. 25 and 37) is common to them all.

Direct infection produces a corneal ulcer or abscess infiltrating the corneal stroma with pus cells or even the anterior chamber with a white fluid level shaped like a hyphaema (Fig. 29).

Continued contact between inflamed lid conjunctiva and the eye frets away the corneal epithelium into multiple pin-point dimples (superficial punctate keratitis).

Ultraviolet light which is totally absorbed by the cornea can cover its whole surface in a similar fashion. An arc-welder is the most likely victim, but winter sportsmen who scorn to use protective glasses in bright sunlight suffer the same condition with the more romantic name of 'snow blindness'.

Now antibiotics play an active role in the treatment of an infected keratitis, but they offer only comfort and protection against secondary infection to those whose keratitis grumbles on, long after the organisms responsible have vanished. These latter respond best to closure of the eyelids (tarsorrhaphy) either long term with stitches or short term with adhesive tape. It is presumed in such cases that the exposed cornea heals with reluctance because of loss of pain sensation or actual trophic changes.

This section finishes with a plea and two simple rules. The plea is that steroids should never be brought near a dendritic ulcer. The herpes virus thrives on steroids, even if they are linked to an antibiotic.

The two rules should remove doubts about how to deal with the pupil of the red eye.

Rule I. If the pupil is dilated, it is safe to constrict it.

Rule II. If the pupil is constricted, it is safe to dilate it.

TRAUMA

Injuries, no matter where they strike the body, have two aspects. The first, and obvious one, is the instant damage; the second is the possible long term complications either at the site of the injury or at a more distant site.

Apart from a few well defined situations that demand urgent specialist attention, anyone familiar with the craft of suturing can attend to most ocular injuries; they are skin lacerations usually, and 'ocular' only because they lie around the eyes.

Now injuries become 'specialist ocular' in four main categories, and the only equipment necessary to evaluate the damage is a good torch, whilst the other eye may serve as a normal control.

Intraocular foreign body

In any violence involving the eye, a foreign body within the globe should always be suspected. Fragments of steel from a hammer or chisel, or pieces of a shattered windscreen are common culprits.

A good routine history should tell if anything was travelling fast enough to penetrate the eye.

Close examination of the eyeball may show an entry point, iris distortion being a helpful guide. *But* should the fragment have entered at the limbus, the eye could look entirely normal.

ACTION

If an eye hospital is close at hand, then referral is the correct approach. However, in remoter districts, a radiograph

of the orbit is a useful preliminary. Absence of orbital
opacities could save a needless journey; whereas a positive film
could save the eye, since early surgery could prevent
destruction of the eye by the metallic salts.

The remaining three categories requiring specialist care
are:

> Direct damage to the eyeball
> Injury to the eyelids
> Injury to the orbit.

However, immediate first aid may make all the difference
to the success or failure of hospital treatment.

Direct eyeball injury

This may be lacerating, blunt or chemical.

Lacerating

Lacerations are easily recognized. It is vital to avoid
anything that might raise the intraocular pressure and hence
empty the eye of its contents.

ACTION

Local antibiotic drops should be instilled.

A sterile pad and preferably an eye shield should be
applied.

Systemic antibiotics and tetanus prophylaxis can be given
last of all.

Blunt injury

The imagination can supply likely agents, but ball games
and fisticuffs must rank high in the list. The front of the eye
may fill with blood—a hyphaema which is recognized when the
turbidity has settled, by a fluid level. (Fig. 29)

If the blow were sufficient to cause such a haemorrhage, it

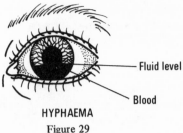

HYPHAEMA
Figure 29

may well have caused a silent rupture of the globe as well. If so, finger palpation will show the eye to be much softer than its fellow.

ACTION

Admission to an eye ward is obligatory.

In remoter districts, it may be justified to delay, provided further haemorrhage did not occur. However, possible late complications call for an eye opinion as soon as possible.

Chemical injury

The range could be bewildering, but strong acids or especially alkalis are becoming popular with bank raiders and have always been familiar on the industrial scene.

ACTION

Instant washing out with water must be the first move with the emphasis on speed.

Complications are inevitable and are discussed in 'The reason why'.

Injury to the eyelid

There are two situations demanding specialist attention within 24 hours:

laceration involving the lid margin;
laceration involving the lower canaliculus. (Fig. 30)

Other lid injuries may be attended to on general principles, but it must be remembered that trauma severe enough to damage the lids may also have damaged the eyeball.

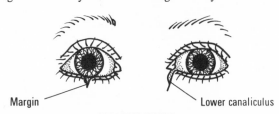

Margin   Lower canaliculus

LID LACERATIONS
Figure 30

Injury to the orbit

Serious orbital damage occurs in two ways.

Fracture of the orbital margin

Palpation should reveal this quite easily.

ACTION

The fractures which are not displaced should heal without disturbance.

Fracture of the orbital floor

The 'blow-out' fracture is one which is not so easily detected. The danger is that the inferior eye muscles may be trapped in the defect in the orbital floor. The tethered eye will not move freely either upwards or downwards, and diplopia will result if lid oedema permits its recognition.

ACTION

The trapped muscle must be released within a week, lest permanent diplopia result from muscle damage.

The caveat in lid injuries still applies—damage severe enough to smash the bones may also have caused grievous injury to the eyeball.

If the swollen lids have to be forced open to permit a glimpse of the eye, a brief comparison with its fellow for corneal clarity and anterior chamber equality may set the mind at rest, at least in the short term.

X-ray examination is mandatory to confirm or refute any clinical impressions.

THE REASON WHY

Intraocular metal fragments

If left long enough *in situ* metal fragments will oxidize, depositing metal salts throughout the eye. Ferrous metals may come out easily enough with a magnet, but other metals like copper would require forceps removal. This manoeuvre could well cause further ocular damage. Despite successful surgery, these eyes frequently do not survive for long; in addition they often develop cataract since the only response of the lens to insult is to go opaque.

Hyphaema

A hyphaema filling the entire anterior chamber can block the drainage angle ('a', Fig. 27) causing acute secondary glaucoma; if not cleaned out soon, the blood may stain the cornea. Later developments from blunt trauma may show up after years. Chronic secondary glaucoma can follow fibrosis of the drainage angle, or retinal tears sustained with the original blow can bring about retinal detachments at any time—so long after, in fact, that the connection may not be suspected.

Acid and alkali burns

These cause lethal damage and washing out is almost always too late. They will distort the lids, causing the lids to adhere to the eye, inturn the lashes, opacify the cornea and scarify the drainage angle. Alkali injuries are the more sinister in that they seep deeper into the eye, causing more complicated disturbance than acids whose coagulating action limits their entry.

Lids

Unless the lid margins are accurately apposed, a notch at the injury site can result in permanent intractable watering not to mention what exposure or ingrowing lashes can do to the corneal epithelium.

The watering which follows neglected canalicular injuries is even more distressing—the more so since early surgery might have cured a condition, which later surgery almost never can.

Orbit

The most aptly named 'blow-out' fracture of the orbital floor can easily slip by the casual observer. The possibly more florid ocular damage or lid oedema can mask the often barely apparent diplopia.

A popular weekend injury, it is often sustained when the victim's subjective awareness is not at its best. A savage blow forces the orbital contents into the maxillary sinus and little skill would be needed to recognize what was what. It is the trivial bumps with slight diplopia hiding behind oedema that the doctor should be on the watch for. Increasing fibrosis can not only make the diplopia worse, but, as the days merge into weeks, it will also make surgical repair futile.

Since many of these cases come finally to court, some attempt at measuring visual acuity makes the medical evidence more convincing, and it may make all the difference to any subsequent damage settlements.

General Considerations

It is to be hoped that the eye is beginning to emerge from the deep as just another organ and not a source of terror. Tissues similar to those in the orbit can be found anywhere else in the body. Skin, hair, vessels, cranial nerves and muscles are familiar to us all. The conjunctiva is a mucous membrane and although tears do not flow in response to food, the tear gland is not unlike a salivary gland. A tear drainage passage can be thought of as a urethra in miniature. Even the optic nerve and the retina, despite its mechanical tendency to detach, do not traduce their cerebral origin. There are only four special tissues.

The cornea maintains its clarity with only a limbal blood supply by using tears and aqueous as blood substitutes. Its deepest layer keeps the stroma free of excess water and disease of this endothelium results in corneal oedema—recognisable as a misty loss of corneal lustre.

The lens relies entirely on aqueous for its continuing good health. A toxic aqueous due to inflammation or uncontrolled diabetes may give rise to opacities in the outer lens layers. Trauma or intense infrared radiation do the same thing for the lens has only one stock response to insult.

The vitreous is the jelly that fills the main eye cavity (Fig. 1). It acts as a shock absorber, but the eye can survive without it if it has to.

The special tissue that need not be transparent is that complex of iris, ciliary body and choroid. The iris is unique in not repairing any gaps in its substance—a quality exploited in the cutting of permanent iridectomies. The ciliary body owes its notoriety to sympathetic ophthalmitis (p. 62) and the vascular choroid feeds the outer retinal layers including the macula.

The management of eye disease demands a little knowledge of how these particular tissues behave, but the principles of treatment belong to all medicine. Any exciting cause is removed; if it cannot be removed, its effects should be mitigated and any disorder of physiology reversed, if possible. Of course in the midst of all this, it should be remembered that there is a patient attached to the eye.

SYMPATHETIC OPHTHALMITIS

A penetrating eye injury can give rise to many troubles, but this condition is its most dreaded complication. In the first two weeks after an injury, especially one involving the lens and ciliary body, circulating antibodies to normal eye tissue may be formed. These antibodies may then attack *both eyes,* which will respond with a smouldering, destructive, inflammatory process.

Clearly, it is essential to recognize the danger signals and remove the injured eye *before* the fellow eye becomes involved—for then it would be too late.

In practice, it can be assumed that there is no danger during the first two weeks when the damaged eye should be settling from the trauma and the restorative surgery. If it continues to settle, all is well.

However, should the eye flare up again, then the renewed pain, watering and redness must warn the doctor to consider enucleation.

Multiple theories as ever conceal ignorance, but it is thought that the injury exposes normally remote intra ocular tissues to the body's auto immune mechanisms and these mechanisms fail to recognise the eye as self.

Although these dismaying decisions are usually taken within three to four weeks of an accident, no perforated eye is ever wholly safe. It is, therefore, wise to regard with caution any casual inflammatory episodes that may affect such an eye.

NYSTAGMUS

The major riddles of nystagmus are for the oculist and neurologist to unravel. To recognize the difference between complicated and simple nystagmus is all that can be asked of anyone else. There are two kinds of simple nystagmus:

Congenital
Endpoint.

Congenital

Congenital nystagmus, starts in infancy. Most descriptions talk of pendular, equal movements, usually from side to side. It is useful to imagine the central areas of each eye searching endlessly for a fixation point that for ever eludes them.

ACTION

Any such situation in childhood calls for referral to establish the best visual acuity.

Endpoint

When the eyes move into extreme lateral gaze, the muscles fatigue quickly. The eyes tend to drift back slowly to the central position, then flick back in the direction of gaze. The direction of this nystagmus is always in the direction of gaze. (Fig. 31)

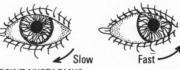
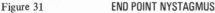

Figure 31   **END POINT NYSTAGMUS**

While normal in the healthy, it becomes exaggerated in the debilitated and, of course, if there is a lateral rectus (sixth nerve) weakness when the exaggeration is on the affected side.

All other uncontrolled jerking eye movements point to some lesion of the areas that regulate ocular motility. These range from the cerebellum to the vestibular nuclei to the brain stem to the inner ear and must include causes such as multiple sclerosis, cerebral tumour or cerebral ischaemia.

ACTION

Nystagmus has entered the preserve of the specialist when it occurs in any position, and is not subject to any alteration with a changing direction of gaze. In the first instance, an ophthalmic opinion is more helpful than a neurological one.

ALLERGY

Iatrogenic allergy is becoming increasingly common in all fields; in the eye it can complicate apparently simple conditions.

Most of the local ointments and drops can give rise to an allergic reaction, which is recognized by swelling of the tarsal conjunctiva and skin oedema spreading from the lid margins beyond the orbital limits. As time goes by, the skin takes on a leathery sheen which gives way later to superficial flaking. A simple history will link the allergy with its allergen.

ACTION

The offending application should be stopped at once. G. Zincfrin (Alcon) will whiten the tarsal conjunctiva. Lotio hydrocortisone smeared over the skin *only* will reduce the oedema and ease the discomfort.

GRITTY EYES AND LID INFLAMMATIONS

This is a common problem, afflicting the middle-aged and elderly. Tear deficiency usually explains the situation in the over forties, but there are many types of chronic conjunctivitis where no ready explanation is available.

Tears maintain the health of the cornea and conjunctiva. As age advances, secretion from the lacrimal gland begins to fail and may not be enough to moisten the eye for everyday purposes.

ACTION

Artifical tears prescribed as G. Isopto-Plain (Alcon) may be used as needed to keep the symptoms at bay.

If there is additional conjunctival injection, then zinc sulphate and adrenaline, prescribed as G. Zincfrin (Alcon) will whiten and comfort the affected eye.

These solutions are safe, unlike the umbrella steroid/ antibiotic combinations of which Sofradex (Roussel) seems to enjoy greatest popularity.

Blepharitis

Simple blepharitis is recognized by crusting and redness of the lid margin, and can be thought of as 'dandruff' of the eyelashes. It is most difficult to eradicate.

ACTION

Elimination of scalp dandruff should be the first move. Removal of the crusts with saline, followed by massage of any antibiotic ointment, deep into the lash roots, should clear up the crusting, as least in the short term.

Tarsal cyst

This arises from blockage of one of the tarsal glands which normally open on the conjunctival surface of the eyelid.

When the stagnant contents become infected, the cyst displays all the signs of a lid abscess and is frequently mistaken for a stye.

Spontaneous resolution may occur.

More commonly, the resolving inflammation leaves behind a hard nodule deep in the substance of the eyelid and as elusive as a breast mouse. Although elusive, it may cause not only pain but visual disturbance as well.

ACTION

Infected stage

Intensive local antibiotics in drop or ointment form (two hourly) will attack the infection.

Hot spoon bathing—a wooden spoon, swathed in lint, dipped in hot water and applied to the closed eye will both soothe the pain and help disperse the inflammation.

Non-infected stage

The gland contents must be curetted from the conjunctival surface.

Stye

This acute infection of the eyelash roots produces an abscess near the lid margin.

Unlike a tarsal cyst, disappearance following treatment is usually complete. Recurrent styes have the same significance as recurrent infection anywhere.

ACTION

Treatment should parallel that for an infected tarsal cyst.

LACRIMAL PROBLEMS

Tears formed in the tear gland wash over the globe before evaporating or draining into the nose via the nasolacrimal duct. (Fig. 32)

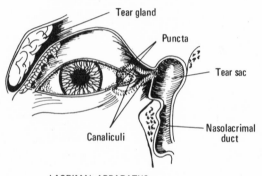

LACRIMAL APPARATUS

Figure 32

The watering eye:

Excess production of tears

Reflex production of tears occur in response to stimulation of the fifth cranial nerve. Thus any of the following conditions will set the tear reflex in action:

Conjunctivitis
Acute glaucoma
Infantile glaucoma (from corneal stretching)
Acute iritis
Corneal problems (abrasions,
foreign body dendritic ulcer, etc.).

Diminished removal of tears
The lids
The lids should contact the globe snugly to allow the punctum access to the tears. Thus in-turned lids (entropion) or out-turned lids (ectropion) will force any excess tears to dribble over onto the cheek.

ACTION
Small plastic procedures are necessary to restore the lid to its former position, but an antibiotic ointment may protect the cornea and conjunctiva until one of these is done.

Blocked nasolacrimal duct (in babies)
The nasolacrimal duct often fails to open fully at birth.

ACTION
It should be assumed that the block is not permanent, and G. Zincfrin (Alcon) may induce free passage of tears. Should watering persist or infection supervene, then probing under general anaesthesia should remove the blocking membrane. It should be remembered that tear secretion begins some days after birth. Therefore 'watering' at birth means infection and urgent treatment is necessary.

Blocked nasolacrimal duct (in adults)
In adults, blockage often occurs following nasal and sinus problems.

ACTION
G. Zincfrin (Alcon) may induce the duct to resume its function by decongestion. If this fails, then it is up to the patient to decide if the symptoms are bad enough to warrant surgery, which would attempt to join the tear sac to the nasal

cavity, bypassing the blocked duct—the so-called dacryocystorhinostomy.

Acute Dacryocystisis

Stagnation and infection of the tear sac contents is followed by abscess formation.

A fiery swelling over the tear sac (Fig. 32) gives the diagnosis without further questioning.

ACTION

Systemic antibiotics should quell the immediate inflammation which however will only recur unless the tear sac is removed (in elderly patients) or anastamosed to the nose.

Acute dacryoadenitis

This rare condition is recognised from all the signs of inflammation over the tear gland.

ACTION

Should systemic antibiotics fail, then non purulent causes of gland inflammation should be considered.

HERPES ZOSTER OPHTHALMICUS

We can all recognize the vesicle to pustule to scar pattern of skin shingles. When the virus attacks the first division of the trigeminal nerve, the basic pathology remains unchanged, with one difference: as well as causing the well-known skin eruptions the infection may give rise to:

Conjunctivitis
Keratitis
Iritis.

The recognition, dangers and treatment of these three conditions, whatever the cause, have already been discussed. Just because the infecting agent is the shingles virus, it does not alter the principles of treatment. Although the skin and conjunctival lesions may give the impression that the whole eye is in the grip of some dreadful infection, the cornea and iris frequently escape unscathed.

Another noteworthy fact is the sequence of involvement, skin, conjuctiva, cornea then iris. An iritis must be preceded by a keratitis, a keratitis by a conjunctivitis, and so on.

ACTION:
A *close* look at the eye with a simple torch will tell just how far the eye has been affected. Treatment then should follow along standard lines for skin, eyelid and conjunctival infection. However, once the virus has gone beyond the conjunctiva, the condition demands a specialist opinion fairly quickly.

PAINFUL EYES

Pain in the eyes can be dramatic and certainly the cause of a good deal of needless anxiety. The starting premise for diagnosis is simple.

If the pain in the eye is caused by the eye, or its surrounding tissues, then the reason will be clear on a direct examination.

The only necessary instrument is a good torch.

The red eye has been discussed elsewhere and the possible causes can be completed by adding:

Tarsal cysts (blocked glands in the tarsal plate)
Styes (infected lash roots)
Infection of the tear glands
Infection of the tear sac
Herpes zoster.

Stabbing pain in the eyes, burning pains behind the eyes, and so on, are familiar to anyone involved in clinical medicine. This is not the place to delve into the differential diagnoses of headaches, but sinus trouble and stress cause far more pain around the eyes than do the eyes themselves.

There is but one condition to be on guard for, and that is the creeping form of angle-closure glaucoma when the only complaint may be of dull ache above the eyebrow. The pupil may be already fixed, but this is not always so (Fig. 23).

LARGE EYES

Large, lustrous eyes are often the most arresting feature of child portraiture. They are also the most arresting feature of infantile glaucoma, but not only are they not lustrous, they are often blind as well. (Fig. 33)

Rising intraocular pressure distends the growing eye to often enormous proportions, but often at a different rate from the fellow eye.

Watering, blepharospasm and corneal cloudiness complete the picture in any infant up the the age of 3 years.

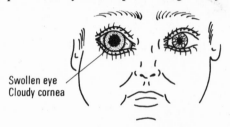

Swollen eye
Cloudy cornea

Figure 33

**INFANTILE GLAUCOMA
(RIGHT)**

ACTION

The cure, if any, must be surgical.

The aim is to clear the angle of abnormal tissue, in the hope that the draining meshwork is itself normal. This hope is not always fulfilled.

Occasionally children and adults have asymptomatic eyes of varying size. Should serious disease be suspected, then referral is indicated.

PTOSIS AND PROPTOSIS

Ptosis

Ptosis, or dropped eyelid, is not a common presenting complaint.

In infancy, the muscle which raises the eyelid is congenitally weak and so also may be the superior rectus muscle which has the same origin in the embryo.

ACTION

When the lid obscures the pupil, the central vision is in danger of becoming lazy. Assessment of visual acuity and, if necessary, continued orthoptic care up to the age of 5 years may be required. The lid can be easily raised surgically.

An additional danger is an associated vertical squint which would reinforce the drift towards amblyopia.

In adult life, ptosis of *recent* onset means usually one of three things:

    Third-nerve palsy (pupil dilated)
    Horner's syndrome (pupil constricted)
    Myasthenia gravis.

These are fully explained under 'Diplopia'.

Proptosis

When the orbital contents push the eye forwards, there are two main dangers to the eye: compression of the optic nerve and exposure of the cornea, leading to evaporation of tears, drying and ulceration of the corneal epithelium.

The commonest cause affecting one or both sides is an overactive thyroid. Thereafter, the well-known systematic aetiological list of neoplasia, trauma, inflammation, etc. will provide an endless collection of possibilities.

ACTION

A lubricating ointment, such as sulphacetamide 2½ per cent, or better still, surgical narrowing of the palpebral fissure will protect the cornea.

Referral to uncover the aetiology is mandatory.

EXUDATES

Like those fragments of history that linger from our schooldays but never quite link up, exudates form part of that ophthalmic jargon we have all heard of but never quite grasp.

There are two kinds of exudates:

Hard

Soft.

Hard exudates (Fig. 34)

Can be thought of as a leakage of fatty, non-cellular blood products into the deep retinal layers. Their edges are sharp and their colour varies from yellow to waxy white. Any general disease affecting the small blood vessels will give rise to hard exudates, and the favourite site is around the macular area. Examples would be:

Diabetes

Hypertension

Angiomatosis.

Any local condition of the small vessels will also give rise to similar exudates, usually more massive in distribution and usually in one eye. One example would be Coats' disease, where the exudates involve the whole posterior pole while lying adjacent are bizarre nodules and vessel complexes.

Soft exudates:

Strictly speaking, these are not exudates at all. They resemble fluffy patches of cotton wool, are evanescent and scanty, and are actual infarcts of the retina which block from the view the choroidal red pattern.

Underlying disorders to consider would be:
  Severe hypertension
  The 'collagen diseases'
  Anaemia
  Embolic states.

Acute closure of the central retinal artery can be thought of as causing a gigantic cotton-wool spot clouding the whole retina and obscuring the entire choroid except at the macular centre, where the retina is too thin to hide the choroidal redness—the so-called 'cherry' red spot.

It would not be a living process without exceptions, and there are two, both caused by choroiditis.

Acute focal choroiditis   Resembles a soft exudate, but the hazy view with the ophthalmoscope, suggesting a vitreous clouded by the inflammation, should give the diagnosis.

Healed focal choroiditis   For all the world resembles a hard exudate. The clue to its true cause lies in the black pigment bordering the white lesion.

GRADING THE HYPERTENSIVE FUNDUS

It seems that everyone except the ophthalmologist wants to grade numerically the hypertensive changes in the eye. While the aim is clearly to produce a convenient shorthand, the result is frequently less convenient. Doctors may remember the numbers easily enough, but they usually forget what they signify. In truth, they are a needless burden on the memory.

The vital thing to understand is the trend of changes in these arterioles, because they are the only visible vessels of their size anywhere in the body. What is seen in the eye is also happening in other vital tissues—the heart, the kidney and the brain.

In childhood, the arterioles and venules are roughly equal in width. As the years go by, the arterioles progressively narrow and fibrous tissue replaces the muscles until we reach the thready arterioles of the arteriosclerotic adult. This is an almost physiological standard trend, which protects the vessels against a rising blood pressure (Fig. 34).

PATHOLOGY

The young adult

Hypertension in the young will produce rapid muscular spasm, and hence uniform arteriolar narrowing. The cause, e.g. a phaeochromocytoma, is usually acute, the blood pressure rise steep, and the effect on the undefended vessels devastating.

The older adult

In this group, a rising blood pressure will accelerate the

ageing process of muscle replacement with fibrous tissue. In response to a continuing elevation, the remaining muscle will go into spasm (constriction) and the fibrous portions will passively dilate; thus originates the familiar sign of arteriolar calibre variation. (Fig. 34)

As the blood pressure carries on the stress process, further signs develop:

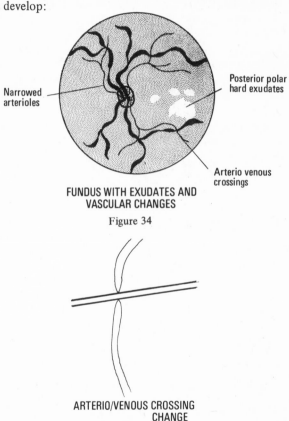

Narrowed arterioles

Posterior polar hard exudates

Arterio venous crossings

FUNDUS WITH EXUDATES AND VASCULAR CHANGES

Figure 34

ARTERIO/VENOUS CROSSING CHANGE

Figure 35

Arterio/venous crossing changes—where the arterioles seem to cut the continuity of the venules. This is an illusion caused by fibrous deposition. (Fig. 35)

Flame haemorrhages   These results from blood leaking into the retina, and the shape is determined by the superficial nerve fibre layer. (Fig. 36)

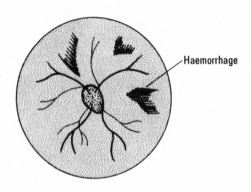

Haemorrhage

FLAME HAEMORRHAGES

Figure 36

Hard exudates   Sharp-edged, yellow/white deposits in the deep retinal layers, usually in star figures around the posterior pole (Fig. 34).

Soft exudates,   Fluffy edged, like cotton-wool patches, random in position and fleeting.

The swollen disc   When this occurs, the patient is in the grip of malignant hypertension (Fig. 19).

ACTION

The presence of soft exudates or a swollen disc indicates severe hypertension. Rapid medical intervention is vital to avoid some cerebral calamity.

In the absence of these two findings, common sense should dictate the management. Mild hypertension is almost 'normal' and treatment of the signs alone is bad medicine. An overkeen blood pressure reduction in the name of treatment may aggravate any existing cerebral and ocular ischaemia, thus substituting a genuine disability for a minor one.

DIABETIC RETINOPATHY

The diabetic retina, like the hypertensive retina, has come in for its share of numerical gradings. These gradings have their uses, but only for the specialist. It makes more sense to forget the numbers and remember that all the following diabetic retinal changes stem from one basic lesion in the walls of the small blood vessels—the so-called microangiopathy. It is important to remember that the same vascular process affects specialized tissue all over the body.

Leakage of plasma results in fatty, hard exudates usually around the macula (Fig. 34).

Bulging of the vessels walls gives rise to microaneurysms, seen as round red blobs, scattered through the fundus.

Vessel closure causes anoxia in the affected retina. Tissue, in search of more oxygen, responds to anoxia, by forming new blood vessels, deep in the retina on the retinal surface, along the major vessels, on the disc and into the vitreous. Whatever these vessels may do for the oxygen supply, they are all likely to bleed spontaneously.

The haemorrhages deep in the retina are round. On the surface, they follow the flame pattern (Fig. 36) of the nerve fibres. In the preretinal areas, they form a fluid level, and finally they may fill the vitreous with floating clots.

Venous distortion and dilatation are currently taken as signs of an unhealthy retinal circulation.

Visual acuity

Visual acuity suffers in two ways: macular exudates harm

the central vision; and vitreal bleeding destroys the clarity of the optical media.

ACTION

Atromid-S (Clofibrate) has a proven use, not only in dispersing the exudates, but also of improving the vision in early cases before the central vision is permanently damaged.

Although retinopathy increases with the duration of diabetes, all diabetics are at risk and deserve regular examination. All haemorrhages excluding the round type, are dangerous and should be referred for treatment, which, at present, consists mainly of light coagulation. The impression is that treatment carried out when the retinopathy is apparently trivial is more likely to have a beneficial long-term effect. The difficulty is to recognize the eyes that are likely to bleed, and although the case for light coagulation is by no means proven, the evidence seems to be mounting in its favour.

A retina that already displays a widespread healed chorio-retinitis (from any cause) tends to escape the destructive elements of proliferative diabetic retinopathy.

The most plausible theory claims that the limited oxygen needs of such a limited retina limit the stimulus to new vessel growth.

Widespread light coagulation produces just such a healed chorioretinitis. This retinal ablation gives rise to disc pallor and narrower veins, carrying less blood—two objective signs of successful treatment. Strangely, it does not cause significant field defects.

Pituitary ablation with radioactive Yttrium can be used in selected cases when light coagulation is not enough.

Its use is restricted to 'healthy' young (under 35) insulin dependent diabetics, who have both lost enough vision and retained enough vision to justify such a mutilation.

Following successful pituitary ablation, although the insulin needs lessen, hormone replacement is obligatory and sterility ensues. Clearly then, patients subjected to this form of treatment must be able to cope emotionally with the demands it makes.

Possibly the threat of blindness may make this increased dependence on drugs seem acceptable, but not all people take this view.

RETINOBLASTOMA

This growth is fortunately as rare as it is malignant—occurring once in rather more than 20,000 live births.

From its favourite site of origin in the posterior retina, it rapidly fills the vitreous with tumour seedlings. These deposits whiten the normally black pupil and it is this feature rather than visual loss which catches parental notice.

Most cases present before the age of three and there is a one in three chance that both eyes will be affected.

TREATMENT

Enucleation is obligatory for large tumours, but smaller ones may be attacked with a combination of radiotherapy and chemotherapy. Both methods can cure a large percentage of these unfortunate youngsters.

In known families, the heredity appears to be autosomal dominant with 80 per cent penetrance. This means that half the children will carry the trait and of this half, four out of five will suffer the disease. Where there is no family history, it seems however that most cases are sporadic and probably not due to a dominant mutation. More and more of these children survive to become parents themselves and their offspring do not seem to demonstrate any dominant hereditary patterns.

NIGHT BLINDNESS

The rod receptors in the outer layer of the peripheral retina increase their sensitivity to light as the intensity of the surrounding illumination decreases. This is called *dark adaptation.*

These rods depend for their health on the retinal pigment layer and the underlying choroid which supplies both the outer half of the retina and the pigment layer.

The night flyers of World War II made the public aware of the relation between a lack of Vitamin A and failure of dark adaptation.

A rather more tragic failure, uninfluenced by Vitamin A occurs when the rods and pigmentary layer both degenerate. This so-called *retinitis pigmentosa* may be recognized in young children, just short of their teens, whose increasing clumsiness in the dusk can no longer be ascribed to carelessness.

The ophthalmoscope reveals an equatorial distribution of black pigment clumps with a shape rather reminiscent of the bone corpuscles of our histology days.

Most cases arise as an autosomal recessive inheritance but dominant and X-linked heredities have been reported also.

The condition is rare, which is fortunate, for it is untreatable. All cases progress from peripheral field loss to total extinction of the remaining tunnel of central vision before middle age.

DRUGS IN COMMON USE

As with exudates, we can all recall, more or less, those ophthalmic medications that provide us with familiar drug names but never quite with their exact pharmacology.

The following list should link the two, and unless particularly stated, local preparations are available in drop or ointment form.

MYDRIATICS

This is the collective name for drugs that dilate the pupil and they all also paralyse focus to a greater or lesser degree

G. atropine sulphate B.P. 1 per cent is the best known. What is not so well known, is its duration of action—14 days, a quality that should limit its use to conditions where lengthy dilation is called for, e.g. iritis.

G. homatropine hydrobromide, B.P. 1 per cent, is the time-honoured short-acting mydriatic, used to permit fundal examination. Its effects last for four days, which is hardly short-acting. It has a very limited place in modern ophthalmology.

G. cyclopentolate hydrochloride B.P. 1 per cent (Mydrilate) is the mydriatic of choice for fundal examination since its action lasts for less than 24 hours.

All three foregoing drugs paralyse the parasympathetic constricting impulses.

G.phenylephrine hydrochloride BP 10 per cent dilates the pupil by sympathetic action on the dilator muscle. It can reinforce atropine mydriasis in severe iritis.

Note   In eyes vulnerable to angle-closure glaucoma (Fig. 28) any sympathetic-like drug increases the intractability of an acute attack. In fact, asthmatics, already frightened by their respiratory distress, may reopen their bronchioles with oral ephedrine, only to find themselves stricken with closed-angle glaucoma.

G. Eppy 1 per cent (stabilized solution of adrenaline). Eppy increases the outflow of aqueous and has a place in the treatment of *open-angle* glaucoma on a twice daily basis. It is of course dangerous in the *closed-angle* situation.

MIOTICS

This is the collective name for drugs that constrict the pupil

G. pilocarpine nitrate BP 1, 2, 3 and 4 per cent is the most widely used. It has direct parasympathetic type action on the pupil constrictor. It also increases the outflow of aqueous from the eye, and so is the sheet anchor in the treatment of most forms of glaucoma usually on a four times daily basis.

LOCAL ANAESTHETICS

The most celebrated and least used is G. cocaine: G. amethocaine hydrochloride 0.5 per cent or 1 per cent has a much wider use. It should be noted that prolonged use of any of these topical anaesthetics can harm the corneal epithelium. In the short term, it is always wise to warn patients against wind-borne particles until corneal sensation returns.

ANTIBACTERIALS

Good bacteriological practice should always preface use with culture and sensitivity tests, but we all need to be practical as well. A wide range of antibiotic preparations is available to suit all prescribing tastes. However, chloramphenicol 0.5 per cent in either drop or ointment forms casts a wide net on both sides of the Gram stain and is a favourite with ophthalmologists..

Sulphacetamide 6 per cent or 10 per cent is a sadly neglected antibiotic, offering many advantages over the others, not least the comfort in application and the price.

CORNEAL STAIN

Fluorescein sodium BP 2 per cent outlines defects in the corneal epithelium, thus adding considerably to the accuracy of corneal examination. The solution has fallen into disrepute owing to its unhappy suitability as a culture medium for *Pseudomonas pyocyaneus,* an organism that favours only one medium over fluorescein and that is the corneal epithelium itself. Clearly, the sterile-strip preparation Fluoret (Fig. 37) is the preferred way to use it. It is also much simpler, avoiding the splashing on the face, clothes and hands, so inevitable with the liquid form.

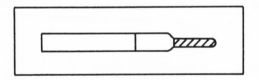

FLUORET (STERILE STRIP OF
FLUORESCEIN)

Figure 37

STEROIDS

These come disguised as a galaxy of ophthalmic preparations, and they all have one thing in common—their danger. If cortisone must be used, it is vital as a minimal test of good practice to ensure a *clear, non-staining cornea.* Mixing the steroid with an antibiotic, such as Sofradex, Betnesol-N, etc. does nothing to increase its safety. If cortisone is going to destroy the cornea neither Soframycin nor Neomycin will stop it.

There are, of course, eye conditions demanding cortisone as a specific treatment but the grumbling, gritty, red eyes that torment us all so often will respond happily to safer preparations like G. zinc sulphate-adrenaline (Zincfrin).

To use cortisone in the presence of *Herpes simplex* is lethal; what is not so widely known is its tendency to raise the ocular pressure, possibly to cause cataracts and to prepare the ground for untreatable fungus infections. It should be prescribed only by an oculist, and then only sparingly.

MISCELLANEOUS MEDICAMENTS

Many people, especially women, after the age of 40, tend to suffer from the 'dry' eye. Now, although sufficient tears may remain for emotional reasons, they tend to fail in their day to day duties. Artificial tears will relieve this failure.

Hydroxypropylmethyl cellulose prescribed as G. Isopto-Plain 0.5 per cent or G. Isopto-Alkaline 1 per cent will solve the problem of the dry eye without recourse to the perilous qualities of an equally soothing corticosteroid. It may be used indefinitely and indeed may have to be.

G. zinc sulphate 0.25 per cent and phenylephrine hydrochloride 0.12 per cent. Best prescribed as G. Zincfrin, these drops are excellent for whitening a smouldering conjunctivitis, and for soothing most other simple ocular discomfort. The watering eye, with partial nasolacrimal duct blockage will frequently yield to Zincfrin. It should always be tried when there is the temptation to use a steroid.

G. idoxuridine 0.1 per cent (I.D.U.). This may be more familiar by the trade names of Kerecid or Dendrid. It is a specific antiviral with a special indication in dendritic corneal ulceration. Since it is antiviral it may also be anticorneal, and carelessly prolonged usage could nullify the treatment by hampering epithelial regrowth.

In acute ulcers, hourly instillation may be effective.

Hydrocortisone. It is ironic that after all the strictures on steroids a cortisone preparation should be included as suitable for géneral use. Hydrocortisone as a lotion has an increasing indication for the skin allergies that follow our medications from time to time. The vital proviso is that it is for application to the *skin only*.

Acetazolamide (Diamox). Although now abandoned as a diuretic, Diamox has an honoured place in the treatment of raised intraocular pressure. The usual dosage level of 250 mg may be given into the vein, into the muscle or by mouth, depending on the urgency. In long-term glaucoma control, especially where surgery is not contemplated, Diamox Sustets 500 mg exercise a slow, continuous curb on aqueous production, and hence on the intraocular pressure. In these circumstances, a potassium supplement is, of course, essential.

Atromid S: (Clofibrate). This drug, more famous perhaps in the large coronary artery diseases studies, has a proven place in treatment of hard diabetic exudates. If given early enough, it may prevent the deep retinal damage that goes hand in hand with long standing hard exudates. Two 500 mg tablets twice daily must be given over several months or longer.

The following list links brand names of drugs with the appropriate manufacturers.

Mydrilate	-	Ward Blenkinsop
Eppy	-	Smith & Nephew
Fluoret	-	Smith & Nephew
Sofradex	-	Roussel
Betnesol-N	-	Glaxo
Zincfrin	-	Alcon
Isopto-Plain	-	Alcon
Isopto-Alkaline	-	Alcon
Kerecid	-	Smith, Kline & French
Dendrid	-	Alcon
Diamox	-	Lederle
Atromid	-	Imperial Chemical Industries

INDEX

Printed by T. & A. Constable Ltd., Edinburgh